The Pregnancy

Cookbook

The Best Way to Get Through

Pregnancy

BY: SOPHIA FREEMAN

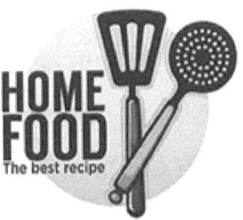

Liability

This publication is meant as an informational tool. The individual purchaser accepts all liability if damages occur because of following the directions or guidelines set out in this publication. The Author bears no responsibility for reparations caused by the misuse or misinterpretation of the content.

Copyright

My gift to you!

Thank you, cherished reader, for purchasing my book and taking the time to read it. As a special reward for your decision, I would like to offer a gift of free and discounted books directly to your inbox. All you need to do is fill in the box below with your email address and name to start getting amazing offers in the comfort of your own home. You will never miss an offer because a reminder will be sent to you. Never miss a deal and get great deals without having to leave the house! Subscribe now and start saving!

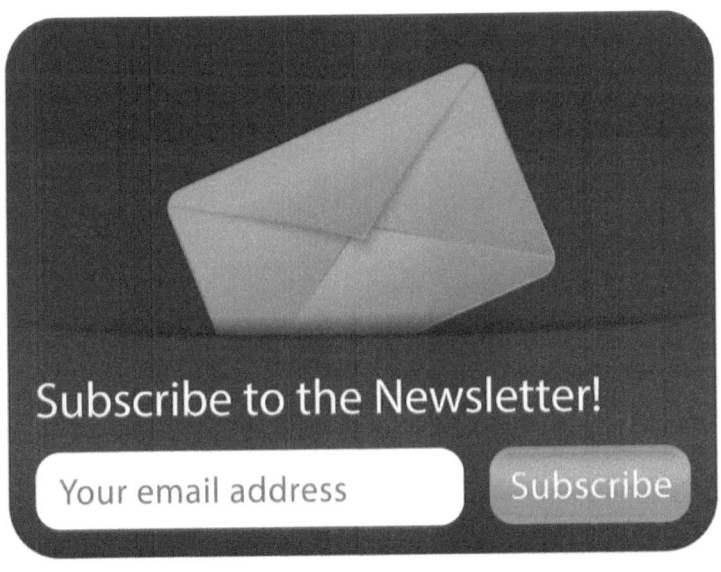

Table of Contents

Delicious Pregnancy Food Recipes 7

Chapter I - First Trimester Food: Should You Eat for Two?...... 8

1) Beef and Black Bean Casserole...................................... 11

2) Greek Yogurt and Ginger 14

3) Spinach & Garlicky Mashed Potatoes............................. 16

4) Raspberry Pastry Delight.. 19

5) Broccoli and Pea Soup with Cheesy Croutons................. 22

6) Tasty Cheese Pasta... 25

7) Smoked Chicken and Avocado Salad 28

8) Healthy Sausage and Apple Casserole 31

9) Feta and Couscous Salad 34

10) Salmon and Watercress Salad 37

11) Tofu and Butternut Squash Salad 39

Chapter II - Second Trimester Nutrition: It Is Time to Beef Up43

12) Ban-pine-kale Juice 45

13) Thin-Crust All-Veggie Pizza 47

14) Oatmeal Raisin Cookies 51

15) Egg Salad Sandwich 54

16) Chicken and Veggie Noodle Mix 56

17) Roast Beef Pita Sandwich 59

18) Spicy Scallops and White Beans 62

19) Tomato Sardines on Toast 64

20) Baked Pistachio Chicken 66

21) Salmon and Pine Nuts 69

Chapter III - Third Trimester Eats: Preparing for Birth 71

22) Chickpea Avocado & Feta Toss 73

23) Vanilla Berry-Green Smoothie 75

24) Hummus with Pita Bread 77

25) Frozen Dark Chocolate Bananas 80

26) Tasty Sweet Corn and Herbs Bowl 83

27) Roast Turkey Breast with Herbs 86

28) Honey-Glazed Brussel Sprouts 89

29) Lime and Mint Chicken BBQ 92

30) Salmon and Summer Veggies in Foil 95

About the Author 98

Author's Afterthoughts 100

Delicious Pregnancy Food Recipes

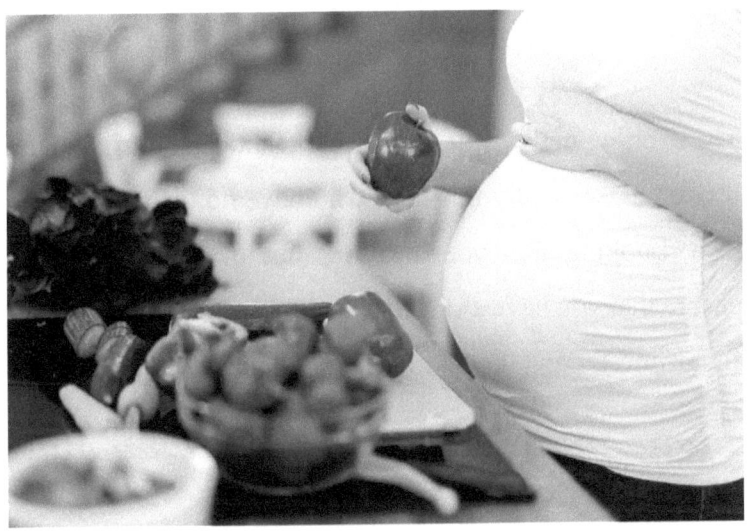

zzzzzzzzzzzzzzzzzzzzzzzzzzzzzzzzzzzzzzzzzzzzzzzzzzzzzzzzzzzzzzzzzzzz

Chapter I - First Trimester Food: Should You Eat for Two?

The exciting news of becoming pregnant can be frightening for some, especially for those who have no idea what to do next. Looking after your health is one of the best ways to ensure that you have a safe and healthy pregnancy from your first trimester and beyond. There is no need to fuss.

ZZZZZZZZZZZZZZZZZZZZZZZZZZZZZZZZZZZZZZZZZZZZZZZZZZZZZZZZZZZZZZZ

Eating for Two?

A lot of women have the misconception that when they get pregnant they have to double up their calorie intake. There is really no need to bulk up; instead of doubling your calorie intake, why not make better, healthier food choices?

According to experts, expecting moms in their first trimester, do not need to add to their calorie intake as the ideal weight gain during this stage is only 1-4 pounds. Instead, they should beef up their iron and folic acid intake both from food and prenatal vitamins. These two nutrients are keys to help ensure that the baby is getting enough blood and oxygen supply to support its development, and that it is safe from birth defects, particularly neural tube defects.

ZZZZZZZZZZZZZZZZZZZZZZZZZZZZZZZZZZZZZZZZZZZZZZZZZZZZZZZZZZZZZ

Ideal Food Choices

Considering appetite loss and morning sickness are not bothering you, these are the food varieties you must try to incorporate into your diet: spinach, nuts, lentils, citrus fruits, broccoli, eggs and lean meats.

You cannot compromise nutrition, not at any moment during your pregnancy. If you are having a hard time keeping down anything apart from water and saltines, try the following tips:

- Eat in small portions.
- Eat often.
- Color your plate with bright greens and oranges.
- Go for whole grains.
- Choose plain, non-fat, less-spicy meals.

Your first trimester is a time to form good food habits that will hold you together for the rest of your pregnancy.

ZZZZZZZZZZZZZZZZZZZZZZZZZZZZZZZZZZZZZZZZZZZZZZZZZZZZZZZZZZZZZZZZ

1) Beef and Black Bean Casserole

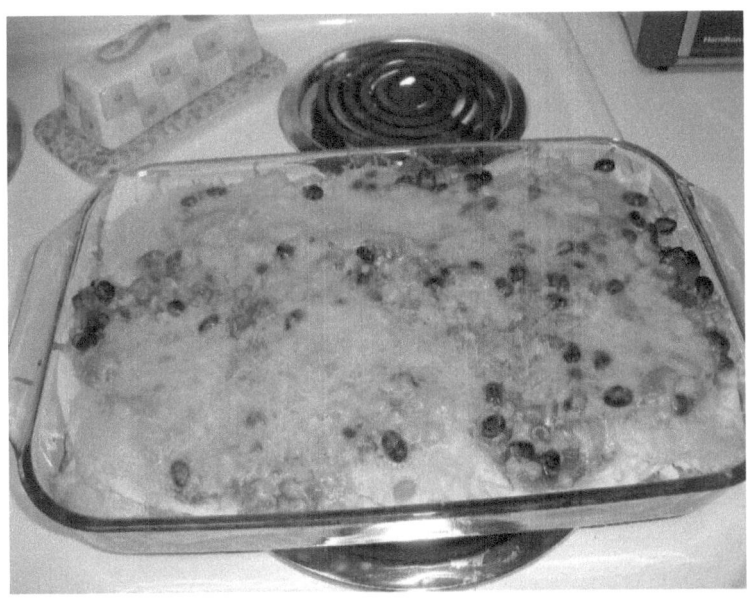

A precious casserole of beef and beans is a great dinner option that moms in their first trimester can indulge in. Its yummy goodness is also packed with a bunch of nutrients, valuable for the growing baby's needs during this early stage. Beef provides enormous amount of protein while black beans have calcium, iron, folate, fiber, and zinc - the key nutrients that you need to grow a healthy baby.

Yield: 8

Preparation Time: 75 minutes

Ingredient List:

- 2½ lbs. stewing beef steak
- ½ lb. black eye beans
- ¼ cup butter
- 2 garlic cloves, chopped
- 2 onions, sliced thinly
- Salt and pepper to taste

zzzzzzzzzzzzzzzzzzzzzzzzzzzzzzzzzzzzzzzzzzzzzzzzzzzzzzzzzzzzzzzzzzzzzz

Methods:

1. Heat butter in a large saucepan over medium-low heat.

2. Sauté onions, stirring for 5 minutes or until translucent.

3. Stir in garlic, cooking for another minute or two.

4. Add beef, stirring occasionally for 30 minutes, or until the meat is tender.

5. Whisk in cooked beans. Season with salt and pepper.

6. Cover mixture with enough water to boil over medium-high heat.

7. Reduce heat and cover the pan. Simmer mixture for 30 minutes over low, until the liquid is almost fully absorbed.

2) Greek Yogurt and Ginger

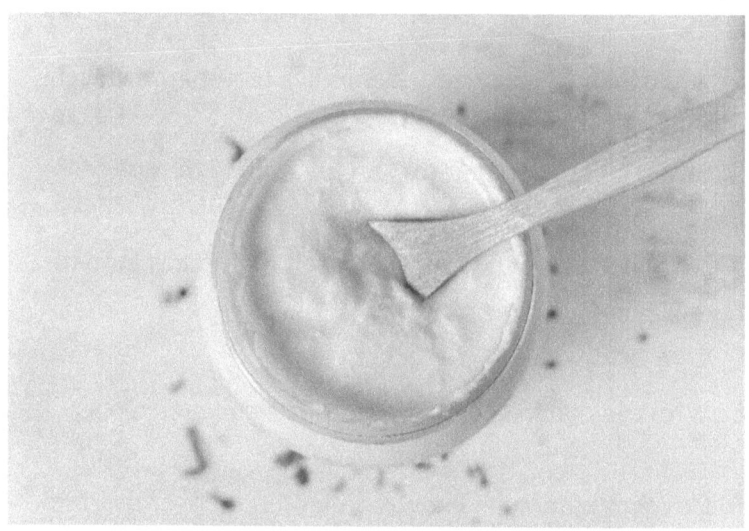

During pregnancy, there are a lot more reasons for you to love yogurt. This creamy concoction can be an another one. Do not choose just any yogurt for this recipe but Greek yogurt, a variety that is packed with more protein. You will need that for significantly healthier fetal development. Throw in some coconut and ginger for a nice, tropical flavor that you will surely adore.

Yield: 1

Preparation Time: 5 Minutes

Ingredient List:

- 8 oz. plain Greek yogurt
- 1½ tsp. coconut milk
- ½ tsp. candied ginger, minced
- 1 Tbsp. toasted shaved coconut
- Sweetener to taste

zzzzzzzzzzzzzzzzzzzzzzzzzzzzzzzzzzzzzzzzzzzzzzzzzzzzzzzzzzzzzzzzz

Methods:

1. Stir ginger and coconut milk into yogurt. Add a bit of sugar/honey/Torani syrup for desired sweetness.

2. Top with toasted shaved coconut. Serve.

3) Spinach & Garlicky Mashed Potatoes

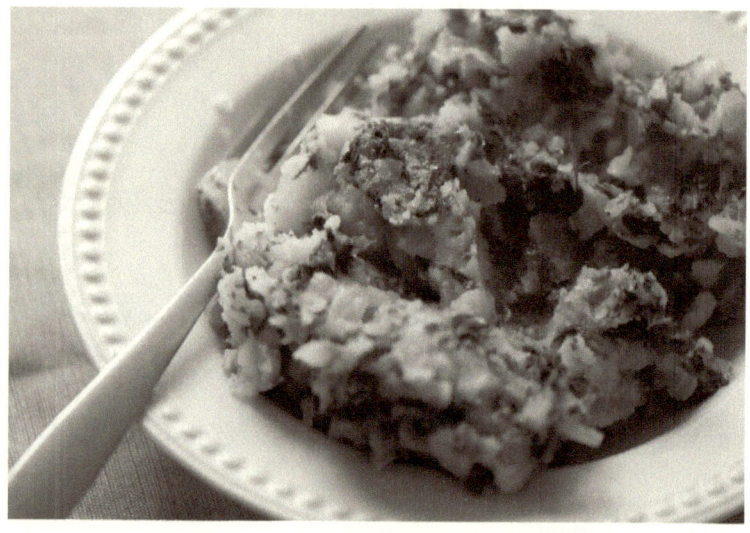

Folic acid is a primary foundation of healthy pregnancy. It is recommended that women who intend to get pregnant take folic acid supplements at least six months prior to conception. This recipe, therefore, is a great meal from preconception to the early stages of pregnancy. It is made with spinach, a good food source of folic acid, and made tastier with roasted garlic, which is ideally prepared one day ahead for a flavorful difference.

Yield: 6

Preparation Time: 125 minutes

Ingredient List:

- 1 bulb garlic
- 1 lb. spinach, chopped
- 3 lbs. potatoes, washed, scrubbed, and cubed
- 1 Tbsp. butter, melted
- ½ cup skim milk
- 1 tsp. olive oil
- ½ cup water
- Salt and pepper to taste

zzzzzzzzzzzzzzzzzzzzzzzzzzzzzzzzzzzzzzzzzzzzzzzzzzzzzzzzzzzzzzzzzzzzzz

Methods:

1. Preheat oven to 275°F.

2. Cut the top of the garlic bulb, about ¼ inch. Place garlic bulb in a baking dish. Season with salt and pepper.

3. Pour water into the bottom of the baking dish, bake for 90 minutes, or until the exposed garlic cloves soften. If time is not an issue, refrigerate overnight.

4. Smash roasted garlic out of the skin. Add butter and skim milk.

5. Cook chopped spinach in a pan over medium-high heat. Season with salt and pepper, stirring until it wilts.

6. Using a Dutch oven, cover cubed potatoes in cold water. Boil, then, reduce heat to low and simmer until the potatoes are fork tender.

7. Drain water but return the potatoes to the pot to shake off remaining moisture over low heat.

8. Mash potatoes, add roasted garlic and cooked spinach, blend until combined. Be careful not to over-mix or the potatoes can be gooey. Leaving a few lumps is fine.

4) Raspberry Pastry Delight

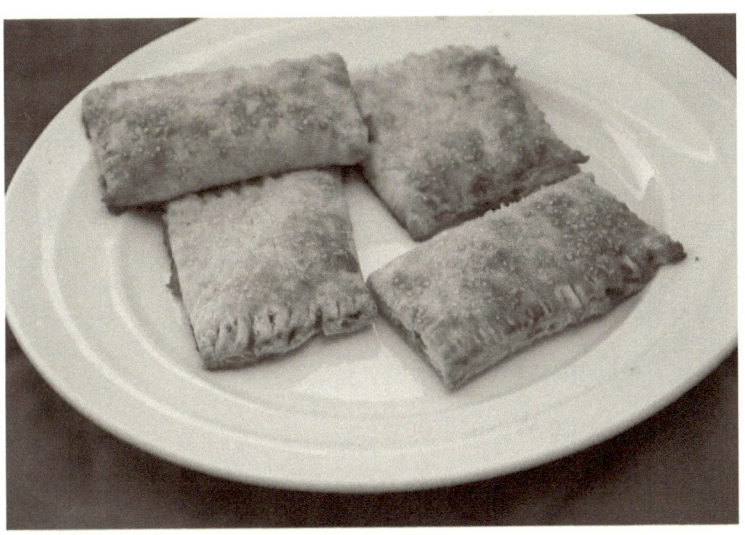

A little bit of sweet is fine, even while you are pregnant, especially if your dessert is made up of berries (which are truly wonderful for expecting mommies). For this recipe, we used raspberries, which, just like the others, are overflowing with unique compounds that offer antioxidant, vitamin supplement, and strengthening of uterine muscles as benefits. Apart from being healthy, it cannot be denied that this fresh pastry treat is ultra-delightful. Serve it with a scoop or two of ice cream and you will be on a roll.

Yield: 8

Preparation Time: 40 Minutes

Ingredient List:

- 12 oz. fresh raspberries
- 1 package frozen puff pastry (17.3 oz.), thawed inside the fridge
- 3 Tbsp. apple juice, divided
- 2 Tbsp. brown sugar
- 1 Tbsp. cornstarch
- For Egg Wash: 1 egg
- For Garnish: Confectioner's sugar

zzzzzzzzzzzzzzzzzzzzzzzzzzzzzzzzzzzzzzzzzzzzzzzzzzzzzzzzzzzzzz

Methods:

1. Preheat oven to 350°F.

2. Prepare two large baking sheets and line each with parchment paper.

3. Heat half of the raspberries with brown sugar and 2 Tbsp. of apple juice in a saucepan. Stir until the berries are tender and the sugar is completely dissolved in apple juice, about 5 minutes.

4. Combine cornstarch and the remaining apple juice, add mixture to the simmering berries and cook for 2 minutes more to thicken the sauce. Whisk in remaining raspberries.

5. Divide puff pastry into four squares, brushing the edges with egg wash.

6. Spoon raspberries into the middle of each pastry sheet, then, fold one corner to make a triangle packet.

7. Press the edges gently to seal.

8. Transfer turnovers onto prepared baking sheets.

9. Brush with egg wash and sprinkle with confectioner's sugar.

10. Bake until the pastry is flaky and lightly brown, about 20 minutes.

11. Cool in a wire rack for about 5 minutes before serving.

5) Broccoli and Pea Soup with Cheesy Croutons

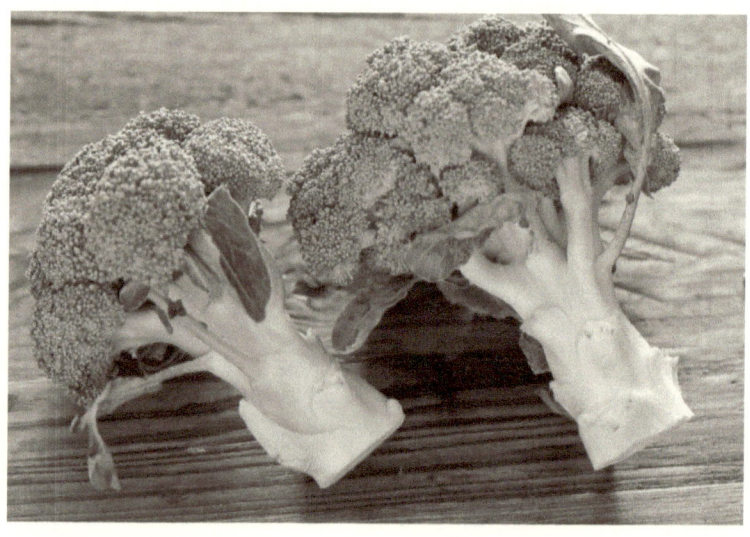

This hearty and healthy soup recipe is all you need to feed your hunger when your stomach won't settle for just about anything. It is light, yet heavy with the right nutrients that you need early on in your pregnancy. It has broccoli, which is a great source of folate and iron; peas, which are high in protein; and croutons made of grilled cheese sandwich, which are ultimately delicious!

Yield: 4

Preparation Time: 35 minutes

Ingredient List:

- 1 head broccoli, coarsely chopped
- 2 cups frozen peas, thawed in the fridge
- 4 slices multigrain bread
- 2 slices Cheddar cheese
- 1 Tbsp. olive oil
- 1 onion, finely chopped
- 2 cloves garlic, minced
- 1 leek, coarsely chopped
- 1 potato, peeled and finely chopped
- 4 cups chicken stock
- 2 Tbsp. butter

For garnish:

- Chives, coarsely chopped

ZZZZZZZZZZZZZZZZZZZZZZZZZZZZZZZZZZZZZZZZZZZZZZZZZZZZZZZZZZZZZZZ

Methods:

1. Heat oil in a saucepan over medium heat. Stir in onion, garlic, potato and leek, until the onion softens, about 5 minutes.

2. Add stock and bring to a boil before adding the peas and broccoli.

3. Reduce heat to medium-low and simmer for another 10 minutes. Set aside to cool.

4. Transfer the soup to a blender once cool and blend until smooth.

5. Place back in the pan to heat through.

6. Preheat a sandwich press.

7. Spread butter on one side of each bread slice. Place the cheddar in between two slices, buttered side out, and cook in sandwich press for 2 minutes, until bread is golden brown. Cut into bite-sized croutons.

8. Divide soup into four bowls, top with cheesy croutons and chives. Serve warm.

6) Tasty Cheese Pasta

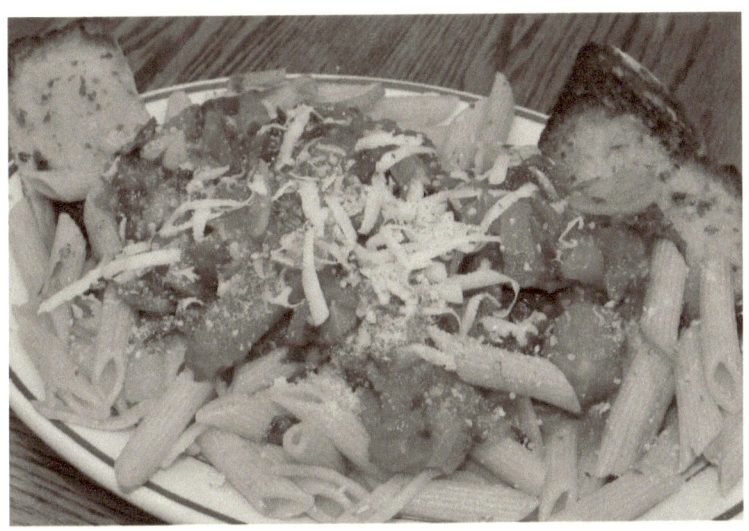

When you are in your first trimester and nothing seems to taste good, you need a certified comfort food that comes with all the valuable nutrients. This pasta recipe is quick and easy to prepare. Plus, it is packed with healthy carbs that you need for your energy supply. It is also a good source of protein, iron, folic acid and calcium.

Yield: 4

Preparation Time: 20 Minutes

Ingredient List:

- 2 cups penne, cooked according to package directions
- 1 cup mixed vegetables, boiled
- 1 Tbsp. celery, chopped
- ½ cup capsicum, sliced
- 1 tsp. dried herbs
- 1 medium onion, sliced
- 1 tsp. butter
- ¾ cup milk
- ½ cup grated cheese
- Salt and pepper to taste

ZZZZZZZZZZZZZZZZZZZZZZZZZZZZZZZZZZZZZZZZZZZZZZZZZZZZZZZZZZZZZ

Methods:

1. Melt butter in a pan over medium heat.

2. Stir in onions, celery and capsicum. Cook for 2 minutes, until onions become translucent.

3. Add milk and half of the grated cheese.

4. Whisk in mixed veggies and herbs. Sprinkle with a dash of salt and pepper to taste.

5. Toss in pasta, bringing sauce to a boil.

6. Transfer to a serving dish, top with the remaining cheese, and serve with a piece of garlic toast.

7) Smoked Chicken and Avocado Salad

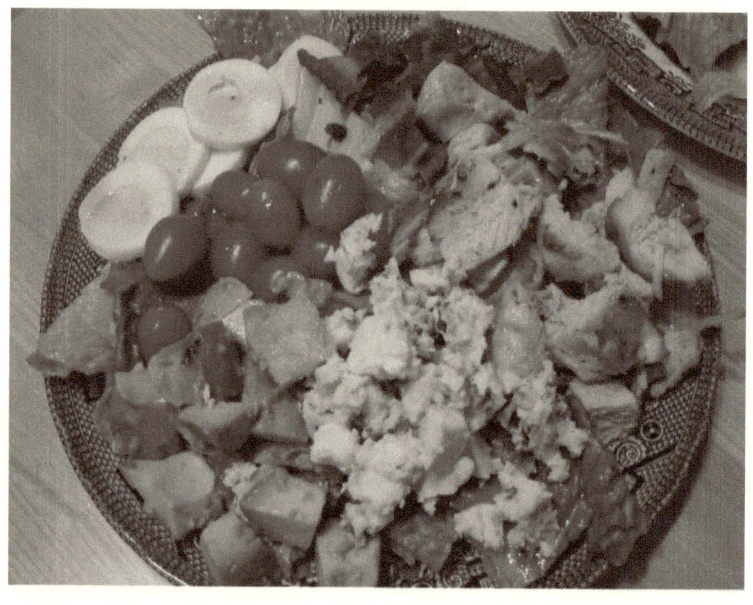

Chicken breast is a good protein source and is almost guilt-free. When it is grilled, oozing with smoky flavor, it will serve as a tasty treat to adorn a healthy salad with. In this recipe, avocado is used not only to improve the meal's texture and taste but also boost its healthy benefits. Avocado is packed with good fats, fiber, and folate.

Yield: 2

Preparation Time: 15 minutes

Ingredient List:

- 1 chicken breast, skinned
- 1 small avocado, peeled, seeded, and diced
- 1 med tomato, chopped
- 1 medium onion, sliced thinly
- 1 Tbsp. flat-leaf parsley, chopped roughly
- 1 Tbsp. red wine
- 2 Tbsp. olive oil
- Salt and pepper to taste

ZZZZZZZZZZZZZZZZZZZZZZZZZZZZZZZZZZZZZZZZZZZZZZZZZZZZZZZZZZZZ

Methods:

1. Season chicken breast with salt and pepper.

2. Drizzle grilling pan with 1 Tbsp. olive oil. Pan grill chicken over medium high heat, cooking five minutes each side until cooked through.

3. Slice smoked chicken into 1-inch thick pieces.

4. Toss chicken with avocado, parsley, onions, and tomatoes. Drizzle with red wine and the remaining olive oil. Serve.

8) Healthy Sausage and Apple Casserole

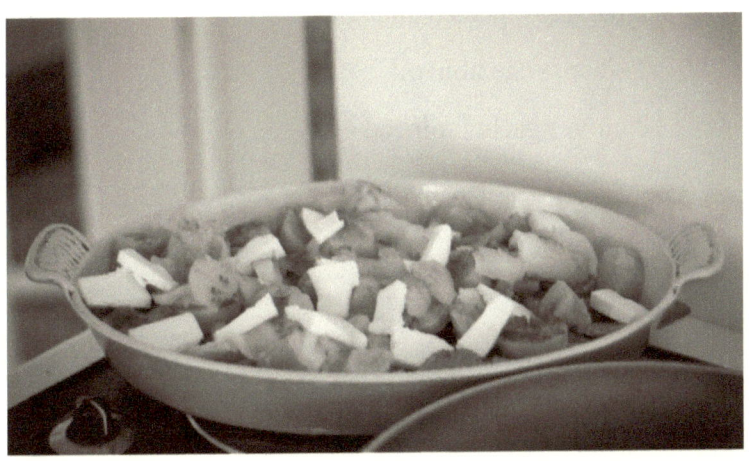

A delicious dinner is all that you need to help you sleep well through the night. This meal is just perfect, with a nice balance of meat, fruit, and vegetables. It's as sweet as it is savory, thanks to a quality choice of pork sausage and the hearty mix of apples and parsnips. Make sure that you prepare enough of this casserole dish to share with the rest of your household. No one, pregnant or not, could possibly resist the yummy outcome.

Yield: 4

Preparation Time: 80 minutes

Ingredient List:

- 1 lb. pork sausages
- 2 apples, cored and sliced
- 2 parsnips, peeled and sliced
- 1 Tbsp. vegetable oil
- 2 cloves garlic, minced
- 2 white onions, chopped
- 1 tsp. flour
- 8 oz. apple cider vinegar
- 2 Tbsp. tomato puree
- 12 fresh sage leaves, chopped
- Salt and pepper per your taste

ZZZZZZZZZZZZZZZZZZZZZZZZZZZZZZZZZZZZZZZZZZZZZZZZZZZZZZZZZZZZZZZZZ

Methods:

1. Preheat the oven to 350°F.

2. Heat oil in an oven-proof casserole dish over medium-high heat.

3. Brown the sausages all sides, about 10 minutes. Transfer to a plate and set aside.

4. Add the onions to the same dish, stirring until softened.

5. Sprinkle flour on the onions to soak up the liquids, then, gradually add in apple cider vinegar and tomato puree.

6. Whisk in the sausages along with the apples, parsnips, sage leaves, and garlic. Season with salt and pepper.

7. Cover the dish until it comes to simmer. Transfer to the oven and bake for 30 minutes.

8. Remove the lid after 30 minutes and continue baking for another half an hour. Serve hot.

9) Feta and Couscous Salad

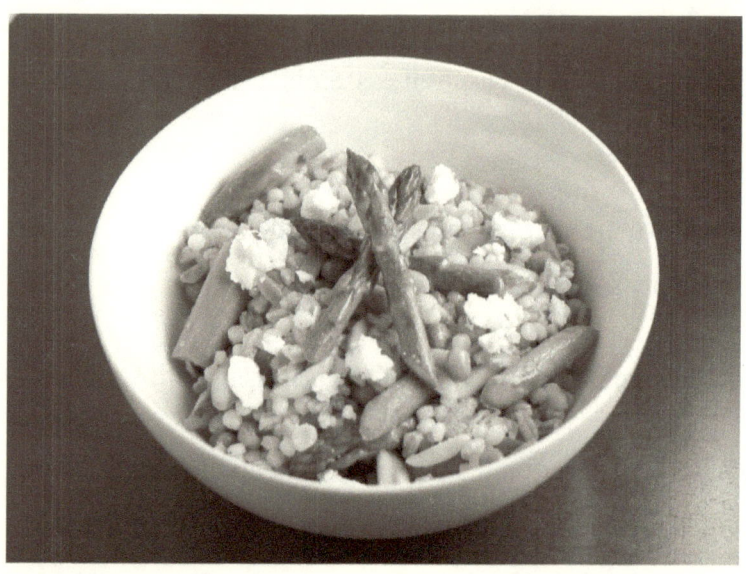

When you have a tough day ahead, prep with a hearty meal that's packed with power nutrients. This salad recipe is perfect for breakfast, or even as a power lunch to keep you up the rest of the day. It is light and tasty, nutty and savory and very, very healthy.

Yield: 4

Preparation Time: 30 minutes

Ingredient List:

- 1 cup whole wheat couscous
- ½ cup reduced-fat feta cheese, crumbled
- ½ cup fresh strawberries, halved
- ½ cup avocado, seeded and diced
- ¼ cup mint leaves, coarsely chopped
- 2 cups arugula
- Juice and zest of 1 large lemon
- 3 Tbsp. extra virgin olive oil
- 2 tsp. Dijon mustard
- 1 tsp. smoked paprika
- Salt and pepper to taste

zzzzzzzzzzzzzzzzzzzzzzzzzzzzzzzzzzzzzzzzzzzzzzzzzzzzzzzzzzzzzz

Methods:

1. Prepare couscous by boiling 1¼ cups water in a medium saucepan. Stir in couscous and cook over medium-low heat for 20 minutes, until the liquid is absorbed. Set aside.

2. In a large bowl, whisk in lemon zest and juice, olive oil, mustard and paprika. Season with salt and pepper to taste. Add couscous to coat while it is still warm. Then, place in the fridge for 10 minutes to cool completely.

3. Toss in the remaining ingredients when ready to serve.

10) Salmon and Watercress Salad

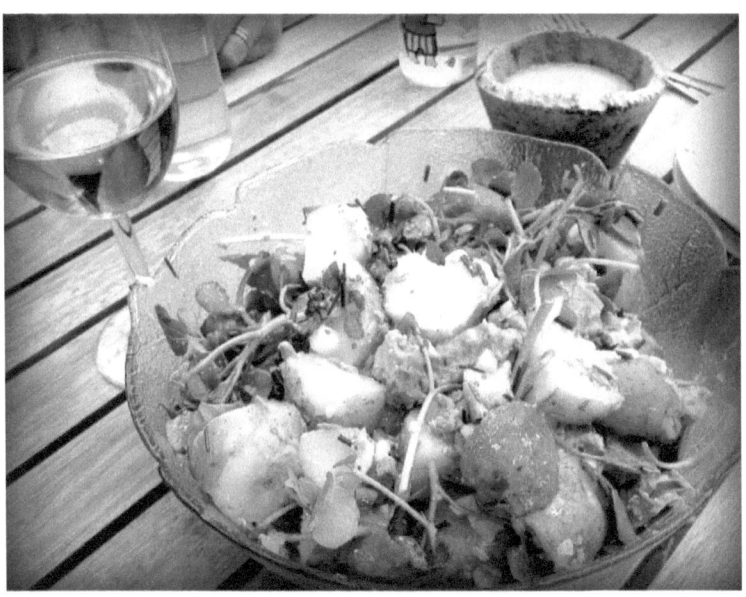

Salmon is one of the healthiest fish that you could turn to during your pregnancy. It has omega-3 fatty acids, which can do wonders on your unborn child's healthy development. As he/she picks up the growing pace, you must remember to nurture your baby with the right food variety. This one is a good pick. Apart from all the health benefits of salmon, not to mention it's delectable taste and appetizing look, there are fresh green thrown into this salad recipe to make it lovelier.

Yield: 4

Preparation Time: 10 minutes

Ingredient List:

- 12 oz. smoked salmon slices
- 1 cup watercress, coarsely chopped
- 1 small radish, thinly sliced
- 1 red onion, thinly sliced
- 2 Tbsp. capers
- 1 Tbsp. fresh dill, coarsely chopped
- 4 Tbsp. extra virgin olive oil
- Juice of 1 lemon
- Salt and pepper to taste

zzzzzzzzzzzzzzzzzzzzzzzzzzzzzzzzzzzzzzzzzzzzzzzzzzzzzzzzzzzzzzzzz

Methods:

1. Whisk together olive oil and lemon juice in a small bowl. Season with salt and pepper. Set aside.

2. Toss all the ingredients in a serving dish, careful in handling salmon slices, then drizzle with a good splash of mixed dressing. Serve.

11) Tofu and Butternut Squash Salad

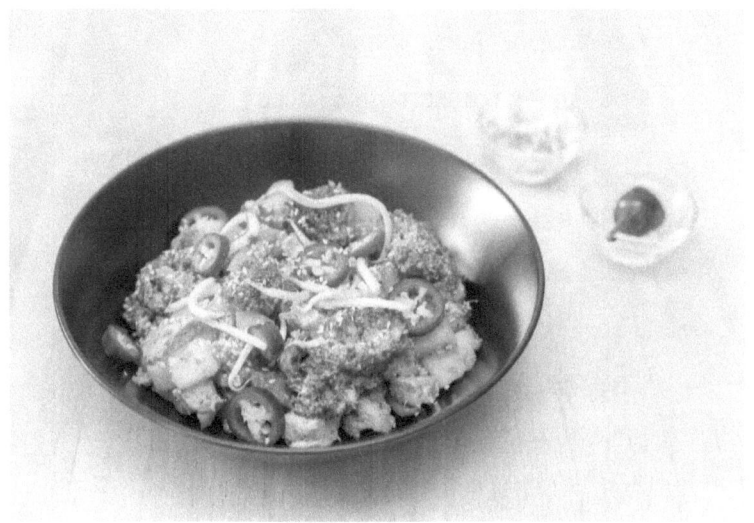

Tofu is a guilt-free source of protein. It is loaded with the nutrient that you need for your baby's bones and muscles yet free from the claws of cholesterol. Plus, this recipe has mushrooms, greens, and butternut squash. It definitely deserves a spot in this pregnancy book as it is packed with calcium, Vitamins A and C, omega-3 fatty acids, potassium and more. Oh, did we forgot to mention that its maple-apple dressing is delightful? Yeah it is.

Yield: 2

Preparation Time: 70 minutes

Ingredient List:

- 8 oz. tofu, cubed
- ½ butternut squash, cubed
- 4 pcs shitake mushrooms, sliced
- 2 cups kale, stems removed and finely chopped
- 2 cups spinach
- ¼ cup avocado, sliced
- 2 Tbsp. walnuts
- 1 tsp. dried cranberries
- 1 Tbsp. cooking oil
- 4 Tbsp. grade B maple syrup
- ½ tsp. soy sauce
- 1 Tbsp. lemon juice
- 1 Tbsp. apple cider vinegar
- ½ tsp. cayenne powder
- Salt to taste
- Cooking Spray

zzzzzzzzzzzzzzzzzzzzzzzzzzzzzzzzzzzzzzzzzzzzzzzzzzzzzzzzzzzzzzzzzz

Methods:

1. Preheat oven to 400°F. Grease a baking sheet with cooking spray.

2. Lay down the squash cubes in the baking sheet. Drizzle with 1 Tbsp. maple syrup and salt before baking for an hour. If you like your salad chilled, you can do this step ahead of time, even the night before.

3. Season tofu cubes with a Tbsp. of maple syrup, pinch of salt, and cayenne powder.

4. Heat cooking oil in a medium saucepan over high. Stir in tofu cubes, cooking 3 minutes per side, until crisp. Set aside.

5. Sauté kale and spinach in the same pan, stirring in lemon juice to cook the greens, until they start to wilt. Remove from pan and set aside.

6. Cook sliced mushrooms in the same pan, adding a bit of oil if needed.

7. In a small bowl, mix together apple cider vinegar, 2 Tbsp. maple syrup, and soy sauce. Season with salt, pepper, and cayenne powder. Set aside.

8. Assemble the salad in a serving tray, combining all the ingredients. Drizzle with the prepared dressing and serve while warm.

Chapter II - Second Trimester Nutrition: It Is Time to Beef Up

Although the first trimester makes all the changes known in an expectant woman's body, only about 10% of baby's growth occurs during that period. For the remaining 90%, the development starts as you enter your 4th month. That makes it a crucial period to mind your nutrition. During this time, most of the baby's vital organs are rapidly developing, so it needs good nutrition from you.

Having said that, it is still unnecessary to bulk up the number of calories you consume. An additional 200 calories per day will do. Just make sure that they are composed of the good variety, taken from healthy fats, fiber-rich foods, and lean meats.

zzzzzzzzzzzzzzzzzzzzzzzzzzzzzzzzzzzzzzzzzzzzzzzzzzzzzzzzzzzzzz

Sample 2nd Trimester Menu:

- Breakfast - Ban-pine-kale Juice, 12-oz bagel with 1 Tbsp. peanut butter
- Snack - 1-2 slices of Thin Crust, All-veggie Pizza
- Lunch - Spicy Scallops and White Beans, 1 serving of fresh fruit, low-fat milk
- Snack - 2 pieces Tomato Sardines on Toast
- Dinner - Roast Beef Pita Sandwich, Calcium-enriched orange juice
- Snack - Low-fat vanilla yogurt

zzzzzzzzzzzzzzzzzzzzzzzzzzzzzzzzzzzzzzzzzzzzzzzzzzzzzzzzzzzzzz

12) Ban-pine-kale Juice

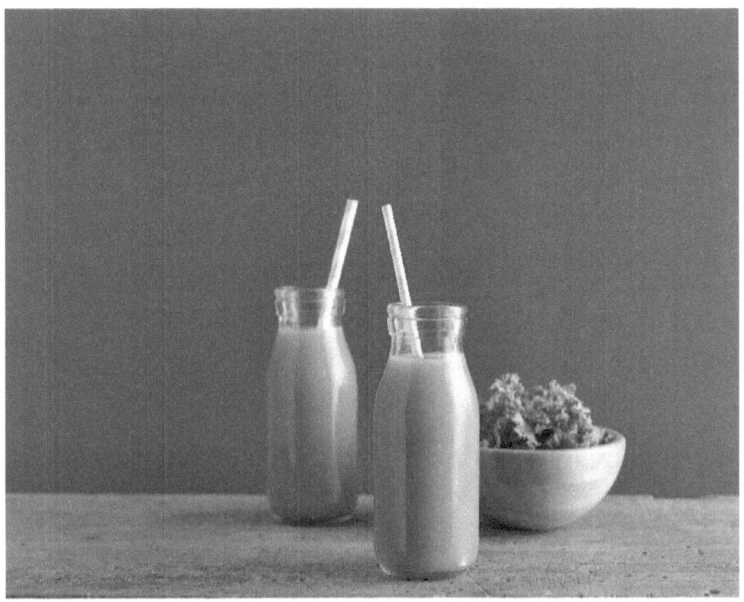

One of the best things about fruit and vegetable smoothies like this one is that you get your dose of the healthy nutrients without having to chew. In this recipe, a delightful mix of bananas, pineapples, and kale provides a tropical delight with all the goodness of greens.

Yield: 2

Preparation Time: 10 Minutes

Ingredient List:

- 1 large banana
- ½ cup pineapple chunks
- 1 cup kale leaves
- 1 cup coconut water
- ice

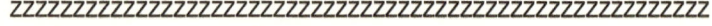

ZZZZZZZZZZZZZZZZZZZZZZZZZZZZZZZZZZZZZZZZZZZZZZZZZZZZZZZZZZZZZZ

Methods:

1. Place all the ingredients in the blender, putting coconut water at the bottom.

2. Process until well blended, according to your desired thickness.

3. Add more coconut water if too thick or add more ice if too thin.

13) Thin-Crust All-Veggie Pizza

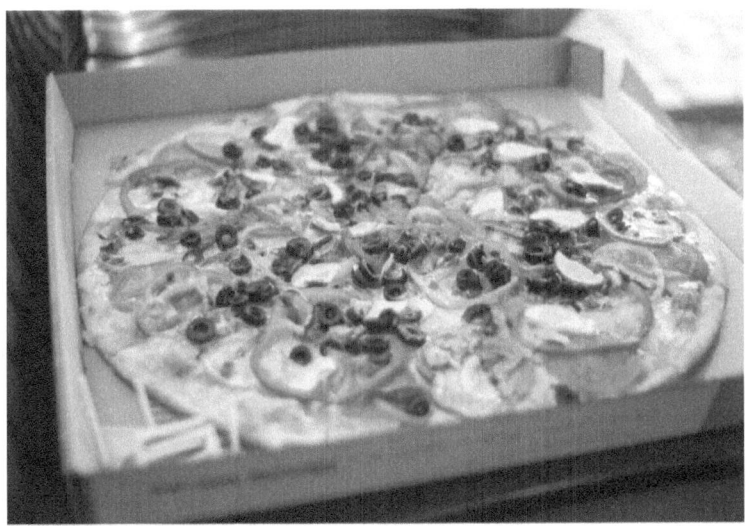

As you enter the second phase of your pregnancy, you need to pack some more calories, from healthy food varieties of course, to support the rapid development of your baby. This no meat, all-veggie pizza with ideally thin crust is not just a joy to make but a joy to eat. It is guilt-free, flavorful, and just perfect for a snack.

Yield: 8

Preparation Time: 35 Minutes

Ingredient List:

- 2 cups flour
- 1½ tsp. salt
- 2 Tbsp. olive oil
- 6 oz. lukewarm water
- 1 tsp. yeast
- 1 red pepper, thinly sliced
- 1 purple onion, sliced
- 4 Tbsp. olives, sliced
- ½ cup mushrooms, sliced
- ½ cup pineapple, diced
- 2 cups pizza sauce
- 4 cups Mozzarella cheese, shredded

zzzzzzzzzzzzzzzzzzzzzzzzzzzzzzzzzzzzzzzzzzzzzzzzzzzzzzzzzzzzzzzz

Methods:

1. Preheat oven to 500°F.

2. Mix yeast with warm water. Set aside.

3. In a mixing bowl, add flour and salt. Stir in olive oil and the yeast mixture, mixing until combined.

4. Knead dough by hand for 4 minutes, until it becomes slightly sticky. Be sure to dust your hands with flour to easily work the dough.

5. Divide dough into four, covering each with a damp cloth, and allowing them to rest for 10 minutes.

6. Put the pizza dough back together and roll out into a 12-inch circle to fit a pan. Carefully transfer the circle into the pan. The thinner the crust is, the more difficult it would be to handle without breaking.

7. Spread ¼ cup of pizza sauce onto prepared dough. Bake in the oven for 3 minutes.

8. Take out the dough, cover with 1 cups of Mozzarella and ½ cup of cheese, then spread the veggie toppings evenly

9. Bake pizza for another 8-10 minutes, until the cheese is bubbling.

10. Allow pizza to cool for at least 5 minutes before slicing.

14) Oatmeal Raisin Cookies

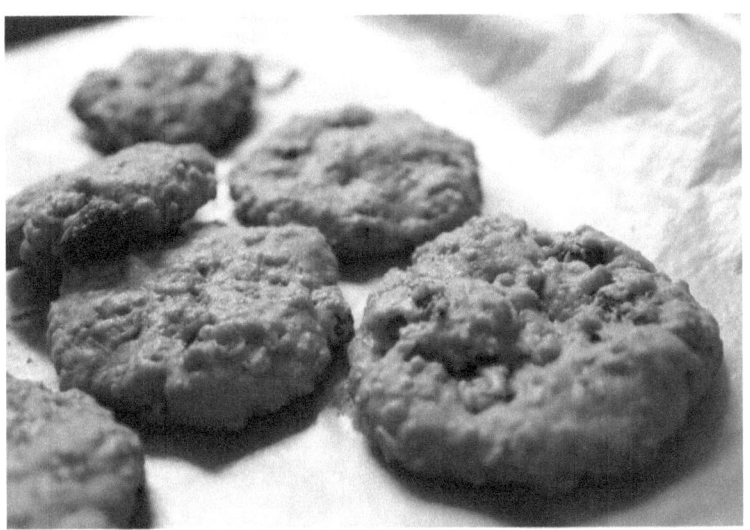

Sweet but not sinful. That's the concept of this treat, so expectant moms can indulge. Pregnancy does not have to be limiting. You must not be constantly stressed, especially about your diet. That's why we included fitting desserts such as this one, in our book. You deserve a delectable treat.

Yield: 24

Preparation Time: 60 Minutes

Ingredient List:

- 2¾ cup rolled oats
- 1 cup raisins
- 1¼ cups all-purpose flour
- 1 tsp. baking soda
- ½ tsp. salt
- ¾ tsp. ground cinnamon
- ¾ cup butter
- ¾ cup white sugar
- ¾ cup brown sugar
- 1 tsp. vanilla extract
- 2 eggs

zzzzzzzzzzzzzzzzzzzzzzzzzzzzzzzzzzzzzzzzzzzzzzzzzzzzzzzzzzzzzzzzzz

Methods:

1. Preheat oven to 375°F.

2. Cream together butter and white and brown sugars in a large mixing bowl. Add eggs and vanilla and continue mixing until fluffy.

3. Stir in flour, baking soda, salt, and cinnamon in a separate bowl.

4. Whisk dry ingredients, oats and raisins into the butter mixture, mixing until combined.

5. Arrange tsp.fuls of batter in ungreased cookie sheets. Bake until golden brown, about 8-10 minutes.

6. Transfer to a wire rack to cool.

15) Egg Salad Sandwich

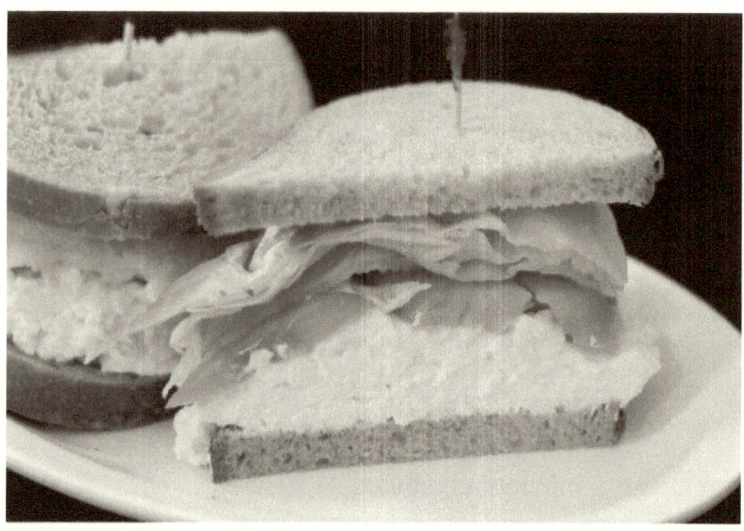

Simple does not have to mean blunt. For this simple recipe, you will get a load of flavors and health benefits, making it one of the best pregnancy foods you can turn to when you have serious cravings. It is filling yet light, flavorful and healthy. It is highly recommendable as a satisfying snack or lunch. You can even keep the egg salad in the fridge, ready for a snack call. Just prepare whole wheat bread and lettuce leaves, too.

Yield: 4

Preparation Time: 15 minutes

Ingredient List:

- 6 hard-boiled eggs, peeled and chopped
- ¼ cup green onions, sliced thinly
- ½ cup celery, finely chopped
- ¼ cup mayonnaise
- 1 Tbsp. yellow mustard
- Salt and pepper to taste
- 8 slices whole wheat bread
- 4 lettuce leaves

zzzzzzzzzzzzzzzzzzzzzzzzzzzzzzzzzzzzzzzzzzzzzzzzzzzzzzzzzzzzzzz

Methods:

1. Mix all the ingredients in a bowl until well combined.

2. Place in the refrigerator, covered, to allow the flavors to blend nicely.

3. Spread on a bread slice topped with lettuce leaf. Top with another piece of bread. Enjoy.

16) Chicken and Veggie Noodle Mix

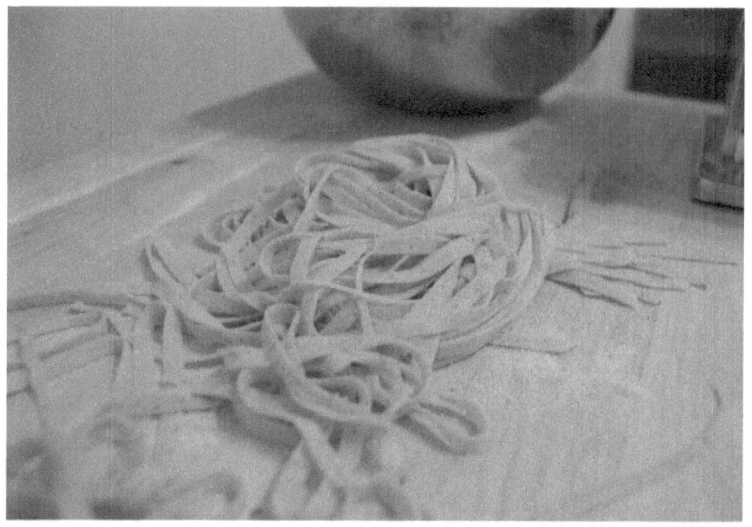

This Asian-flavored chicken is oozing with great things that every one, pregnant or not, could take advantage of. Aside from protein-packed, fat-free chicken breasts, there are veggies and buckwheat noodles thrown in, which made it even more delicious and healthy at the same time. What's more? You can prepare this in 3 easy steps.

Yield: 6

Preparation Time: 10 Minutes

Ingredient List:

- 1 lb. chicken breast tenders, cut into bite-sized pieces
- 1 package buckwheat noodles (12-oz), prepared according to package directions
- 1 tsp. fresh ginger, peeled and grated
- 1 clove garlic, minced
- 2 large zucchini, julienned
- 1 large carrot, julienned
- 1 red bell pepper, julienned
- 1 Tbsp. canola oil
- ½ cup chicken broth
- 3 Tbsp. soy sauce
- 2 Tbsp. oyster sauce
- 2 Tbsp. mirin
- 1 tsp. Sriracha
- 1 Tbsp. sesame seeds, toasted
- For garnishing: coriander leaves, roughly chopped

ZZZZZZZZZZZZZZZZZZZZZZZZZZZZZZZZZZZZZZZZZZZZZZZZZZZZZZZZZZZZZZZZZZZZ

Methods:

1. Heat canola oil in a large skillet over medium high. Sauté garlic, ginger and bite-sized chicken pieces in oil. Stir constantly for about 5 minutes.

2. Add chicken broth, soy sauce, oyster sauce, mirin and Sriracha.

3. Stir in vegetables and noodles, cooking for 3 minutes until well combined. Sprinkle with sesame seeds and coriander leaves. Serve.

17) Roast Beef Pita Sandwich

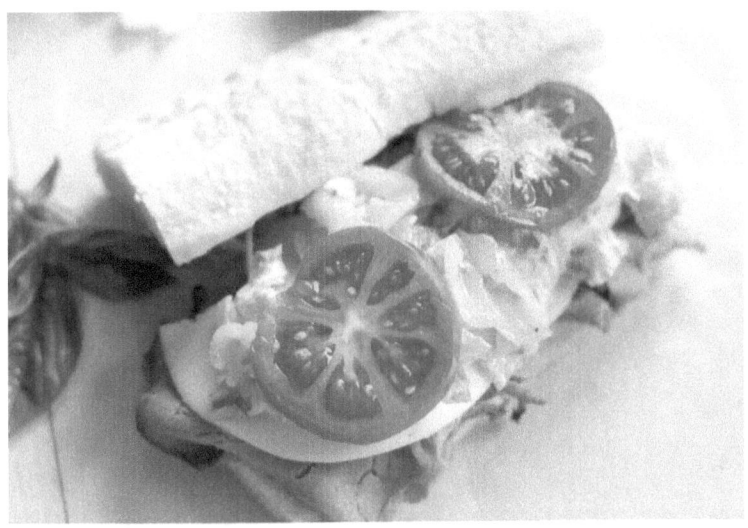

Delectable roast beef is the main feature of this sandwich meal. It provides a rich flavor that's wonderfully enhanced by a creamy sauce. On a health note, this protein packed meal is just the kind of nourishment that you need as you tackle the strain in your back, the hips and everywhere else, thanks to your growing bump. And yes, you will need that protein boost for your little one's healthy growth of strong bones and muscles.

Yield: 6

Preparation Time: 15 minutes

Ingredient List:

- 1 lb. deli roast beef, shaved
- 1 cup onion rings
- 2 pcs tomatoes, chopped
- 1 Tbsp. prepared horseradish
- 1 Tbsp. butter
- 6 oz. cream cheese, cubed
- ½ cup milk
- 2 cups shredded lettuce
- 6 pita breads, cut in half to make pockets

ZZZZZZZZZZZZZZZZZZZZZZZZZZZZZZZZZZZZZZZZZZZZZZZZZZZZZZZZZZZZZZZZ

Methods:

1. Heat butter over medium fire. Add onions, stirring until crisp yet softened.

2. Whisk in cream cheese and milk, stirring until the cheese melts and the sauce is well blended.

3. Remove sauce from heat before adding horseradish.

4. Fill pita pockets with a mixture of roast beef, lettuce and tomatoes.

5. Drizzle with creamy horseradish sauce.

18) Spicy Scallops and White Beans

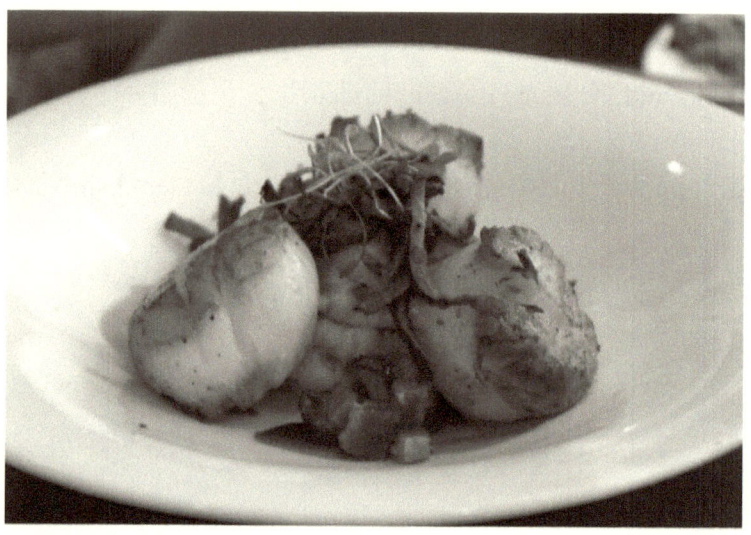

One plate meals are ideal for pregnant moms. For one, they prepare in one go. For another, they will have all the necessary nutrients that expectant women's changing body actually needs. Every spoonful is amazing because it's a spoonful of health for you and the growing lil' one inside of you. That's exactly what this dish is all about. It is very easy to prepare and very yummy to eat.

Yield: 4

Preparation Time: 20 Minutes

Ingredient List:

- 1½ lbs. scallops
- 1 can white beans (15-oz), drained
- 1 big red pepper, cored, seeded, roasted, and sliced thinly
- 1 jar salsa (15-o)
- 3 strips bacon, diced
- Salt and pepper to taste

zzzzzzzzzzzzzzzzzzzzzzzzzzzzzzzzzzzzzzzzzzzzzzzzzzzzzzzzzzzzzz

Methods:

1. Heat bacon in a large non-stick pan over medium fire, stirring occasionally, for 3 minutes.

2. Stir in salsa, roasted peppers and beans. Cover, turn heat to low and keep cook for 10 minutes.

3. Add scallops. Season with salt and pepper. Continue cooking for another 2 minutes. Serve.

19) Tomato Sardines on Toast

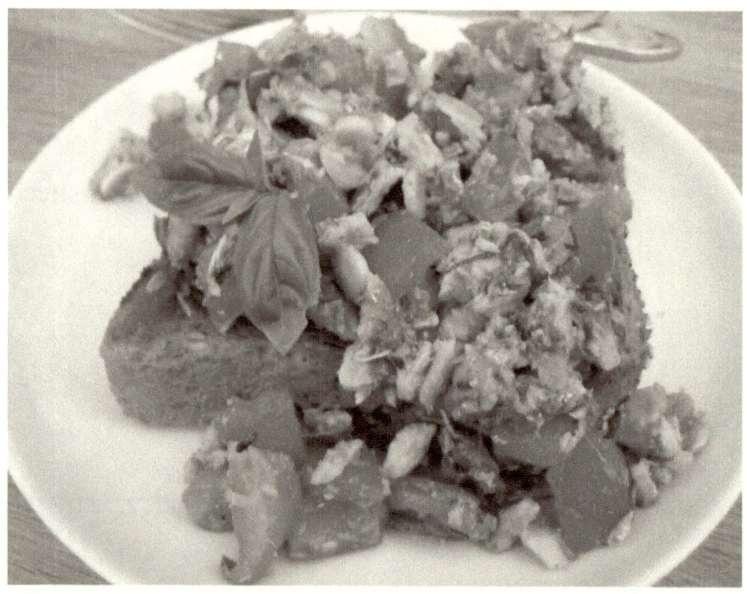

Did you know that sardines are some of the healthiest fish where expectant moms can find a good amount of nourishment? Well, that's no joke. Sardines will make a good meal for you and your baby. Since it is canned, ready at the pantry anytime, you will not need too much effort preparing a good meal for yourself, even when your body seems heavy with all the physical challenges of pregnancy.

Yield: 4

Preparation Time: 5 minutes

Ingredient List:

- 4 tins tomato sardines
- 4 pcs. Tomatoes, sliced
- 8 slices white bread

zzzzzzzzzzzzzzzzzzzzzzzzzzzzzzzzzzzzzzzzzzzzzzzzzzzzzzzzzzzzzzz

Methods:

1. Transfer sardines in a bowl. Break fish coarsely with a fork. Set aside.

2. Toast bread slices until light brown, about 2 minutes.

3. Spoon sardines onto each bread slice and top with sliced tomatoes. Serve warm.

20) Baked Pistachio Chicken

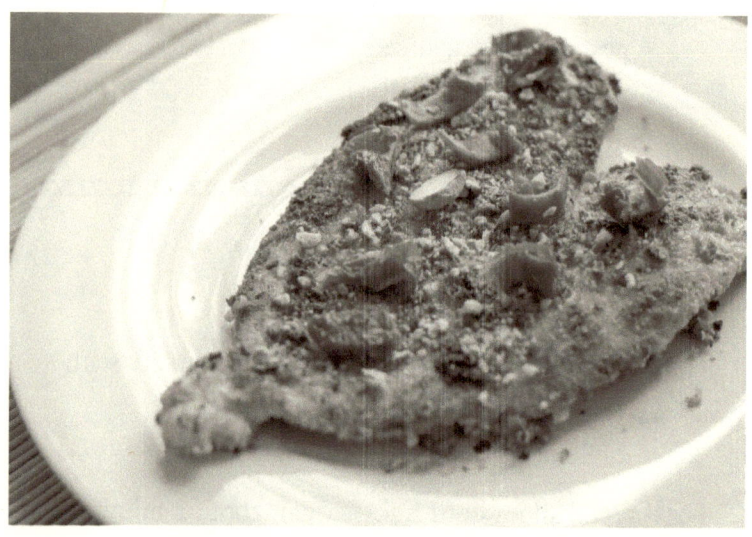

A delightfully crusted chicken with a significantly unique add-on ingredient: pistachio nuts. The yummy source of protein is carefully enhanced by the nutrients that pistachio comes with. Then, there's the fact that this meal is so easy to prepare. You will be ready with a filling meal in less than an hour. Much of that time is spent waiting by the oven, either downing yourself in a fun pregnancy book or another fun activity.

Yield: 4

Preparation Time: 35 Minutes

Ingredient List:

- 4 pcs boneless chicken breasts
- 2 cups unsalted pistachios, shelled and roughly chopped
- ½ tsp. garlic powder
- ½ tsp. onion powder
- ½ tsp. paprika
- Cooking spray
- Salt and pepper to taste

zzzzzzzzzzzzzzzzzzzzzzzzzzzzzzzzzzzzzzzzzzzzzzzzzzzzzzzzzzzzzzzz

Methods:

1. Preheat oven to 400°F.

2. Set a roasting rack over a baking sheet. Lightly grease with some cooking spray. Set aside.

3. Combine chopped pistachios with seasonings until well blended.

4. Press down each boneless chicken piece onto pistachio mixture to coat fully and evenly.

5. Arrange pistachio-coated chicken to the roasting rack. Bake in the oven for 20-25 minutes, until the internal temperature of the chicken reaches 160°F.

21) Salmon and Pine Nuts

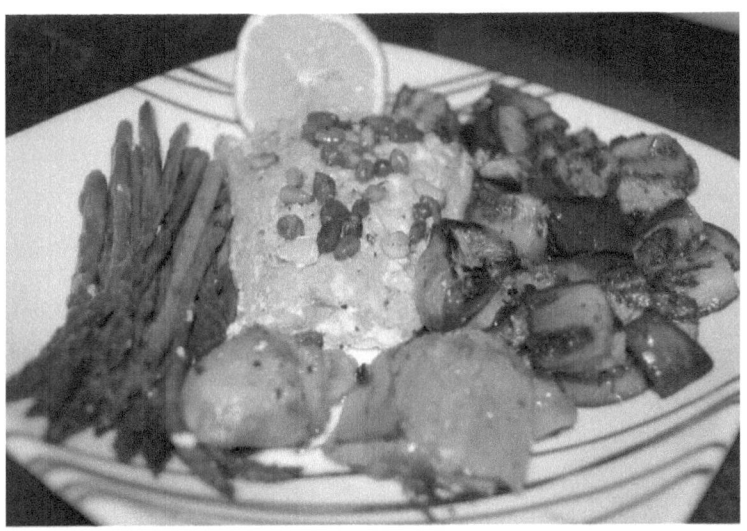

Fragrant and rich, this fresh salmon recipe will make you look at fish differently. It is no longer just about nutrition, but more about a delicious meal that you deserve, considering all the things - changes in your body, mood swings, aches and pains - that you are going through now that you are pregnant. This recipe is truly, one for the books.

Yield: 4

Preparation Time: 10 Minutes

Ingredient List:

- 4 pieces salmon fillet (12 oz.), skin on
- ¼ cup pine nuts, chopped
- 2 cloves garlic, minced
- 2 Tbsp. olive oil
- Zest of 1 lemon
- ½ cup flat-leaf parsley, roughly chopped
- Salt and pepper to taste

zzzzzzzzzzzzzzzzzzzzzzzzzzzzzzzzzzzzzzzzzzzzzzzzzzzzzzzzzzzzzzzzzzz

Methods:

1. Preheat oven to 425°F. prepare a baking tray lined with parchment paper.

2. Arrange salmon fillet on the baking tray, skin side down. Sprinkle with salt and pepper to taste.

3. Toss parsley, lemon zest, olive oil, garlic, and pine nuts in a bowl. Scatter over salmon fillets.

4. Bake for 8-10 minutes or until the fish is opaque and flaky.

5. Rest for 5 minutes before serving.

Chapter III - Third Trimester Eats: Preparing for Birth

As you get near your due date, you are required to stock up energy so your body will be able to ace the challenge. Apart from prenatal supplements, food is your best friend in battling pregnancy fatigue and preparing for a healthy delivery. Eating healthy has a lot to do with feeling good and feeling good will help boost your stamina so you can keep up with the physical demands of giving birth.

Apart from eating for your strength, food will also play some crucial roles on how well the developing baby is growing inside you. During the third trimester, your baby needs protein, omega-3 fatty acids, choline and healthy fats.

At this point, your baby's brain as well as his muscles and tissues are developing oh, so quickly. That's why they need an enormous supply of the required nutrients to keep up. Thanks to you, your baby shall be able to access the healthy vitamins and minerals he/she needs to come out into the world healthy.

ZZZZZZZZZZZZZZZZZZZZZZZZZZZZZZZZZZZZZZZZZZZZZZZZZZZZZZZZZZZZZZ

3rd Trimester Food Ideas

Some of the delectable and incredibly healthy food varieties that you must have during the third trimester include:

- Porridge with reduced-fat milk and fruits
- Fresh fruit shakes or coolers
- Chickpeas and rice
- Whole wheat toasts
- Dried fruits and nuts
- Hummus and pita bread
- Beetroot and spinach soups or salads
- Sweet corn

ZZZZZZZZZZZZZZZZZZZZZZZZZZZZZZZZZZZZZZZZZZZZZZZZZZZZZZZZZZZZZZZZ

22) Chickpea Avocado & Feta Toss

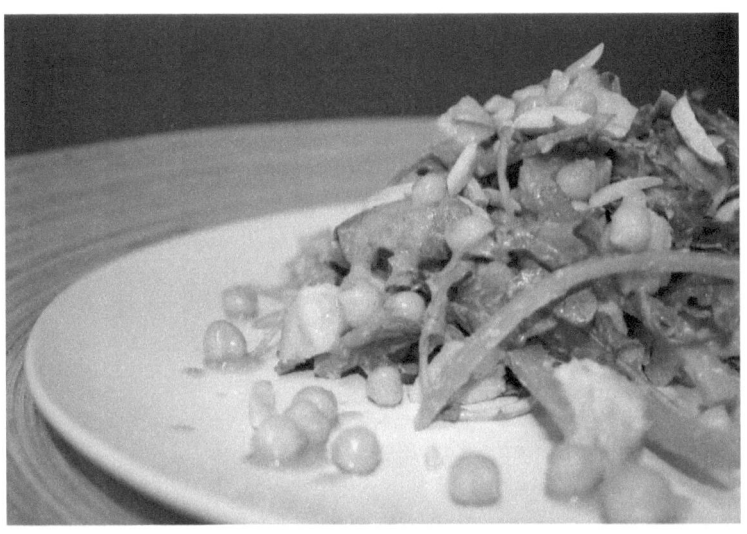

Eating healthy, clean and hearty vegetables is a great way to prepare for motherhood. In this salad recipe, you get a combination of protein, vitamin C, beta-carotene, fiber, potassium, magnesium, and vitamin K. It's a great boost to alter the unhealthy effects of hormonal changes on the skin. Plus, it provides all the nourishment your baby needs to come out healthy and strong.

Yield: 4

Preparation Time: 15 minutes

Ingredient List:

- 1 can chickpeas (19-oz.), drained
- 1 avocado, peeled, seeded, and diced
- ½ cucumber, chopped
- 4 green onions, chopped
- ¼ cup parsley, chopped
- Juice of 1 lime
- 1 Tbsp. extra virgin olive oil
- ¼ cup feta cheese, crumbled
- Salt and pepper to taste

zzzzzzzzzzzzzzzzzzzzzzzzzzzzzzzzzzzzzzzzzzzzzzzzzzzzzzzzzzzzzzzzzzzzz

Methods:

1. Combine all the ingredients in a bowl. Toss carefully.
Serve.

23) Vanilla Berry-Green Smoothie

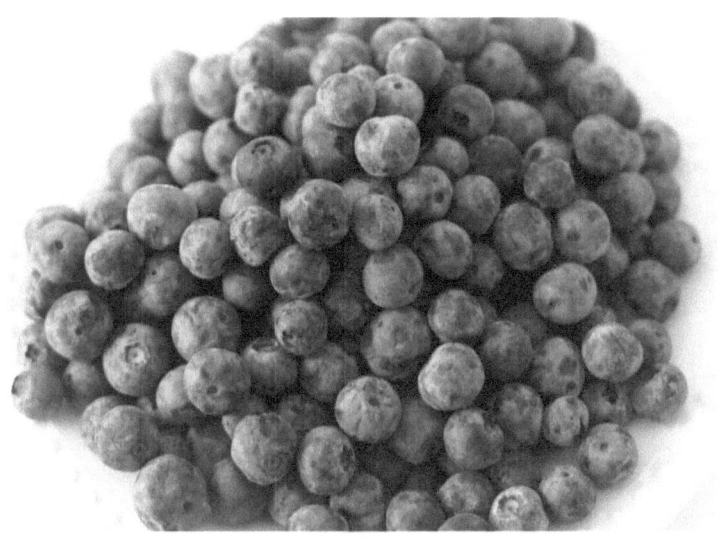

Berries, of all shapes and sizes, are good for your expectant moms. They are packed with all the essential nutrients needed so your unborn baby grows healthy skin cells and stronger immune system. That's why we decided to include a delightful berry smoothie in this book. It's creamy, friendly to the stomach, easy to prepare and utterly delicious. But wait, there's more. This recipe also includes bananas, oats, and spinach leaves, which are great sources of pregnancy nourishment. You can choose to make this smoothie ahead and store in the freezer so you can have a refreshing treat ready anytime.

Yield: 2

Preparation Time: 5 Minutes

Ingredient List:

- ½ cup frozen raspberries
- ½ cup frozen blueberries
- 1 ripe banana
- 1 cup spinach leaves
- 2 Tbsp. oats
- ½ cup milk
- 1 cup shaved ice
- Sugar to taste

zzzzzzzzzzzzzzzzzzzzzzzzzzzzzzzzzzzzzzzzzzzzzzzzzzzzzzzzzzzzzzzz

Methods:

1. Combine all the ingredients in a blender. Process until smooth.

24) Hummus with Pita Bread

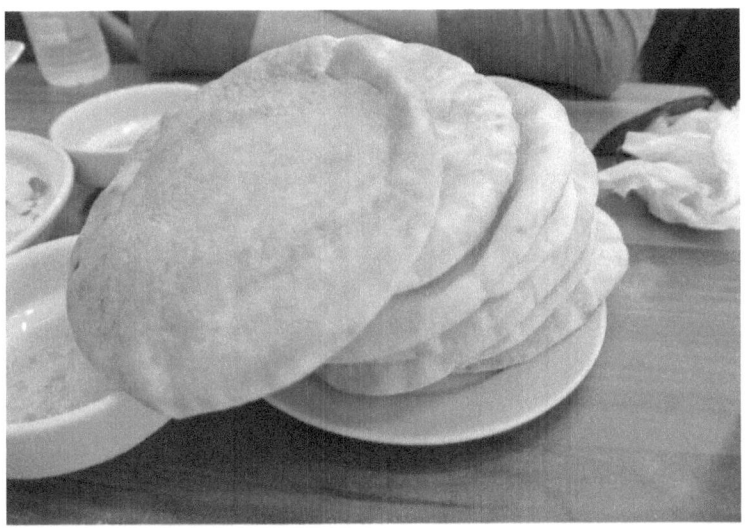

Hummus is very healthy. It has good fatty acids, protein, vitamins, minerals and carbohydrates. That's probably one of the reasons why the recipe, though originally from the Middle East, has America and Europe under its spell. It is a great pregnancy food too, with its enormous supply of plant-based protein and bone-building nutrients. Bone loss is a common concern among pregnant women who have had significant hormonal shifts and a serving of hummus can help address that.

Yield: 6

Preparation Time: 35 minutes

Ingredient List:

- 2 cups canned chickpeas, drained
- 3 Tbsp. tahini
- 3 Tbsp. lemon juice
- 3 Tbsp. garlic oil
- ¼ tsp. cayenne pepper
- 6 pita breads
- Salt to taste
- 1 tsp. flat-leaf parsley, chopped

zzzzzzzzzzzzzzzzzzzzzzzzzzzzzzzzzzzzzzzzzzzzzzzzzzzzzzzzzzzzzzzzzz

Methods:

1. Process chickpeas, tahini, garlic oil, lemon juice, cayenne pepper and salt until smooth. Stir in additional chickpea liquid to loosen up the mixture.

2. Season with salt and additional lemon juice to taste. Transfer in a covered bowl and place in the refrigerator.

3. Grill pita breads over medium fire. Wait for grill marks to appear.

4. Cut grilled pita bread onto wedges. Serve with hummus.

25) Frozen Dark Chocolate Bananas

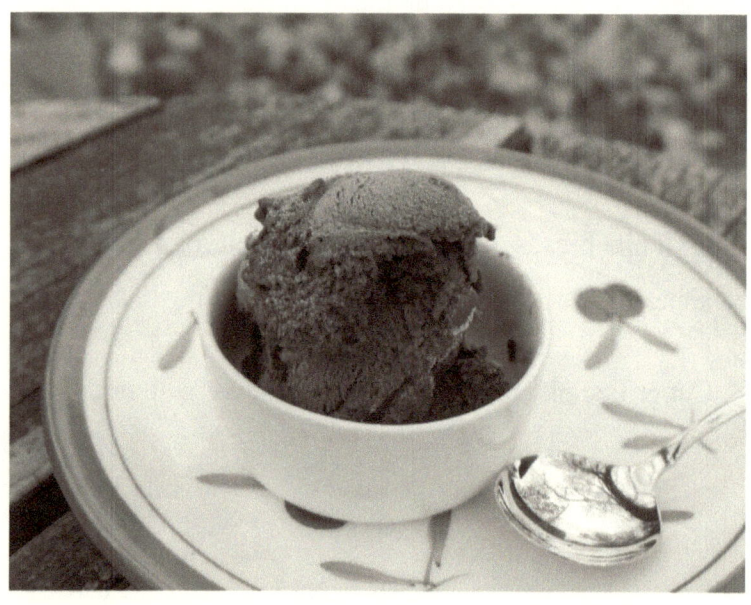

Looking for a refreshing cold dessert that's sweet but guilt-free? Indulge on this frozen banana recipe and give in to your cravings. Bananas are great from pregnant women. It's a wealth of folic acid, iron, protein, Vitamin C, Vitamin B6, calcium and of course, potassium. It can help aid in your digestion. Best of all, it can instantly boost your energy. That makes bananas an ally for those in their third trimester of pregnancy.

Yield: 6

Preparation Time: 172 minutes

Ingredient List:

- 3 bananas, cut into 1-inch slices
- 5 oz. dark chocolate, finely chopped
- 2 tsp. coconut oil
- 2 Tbsp. toasted almonds, chopped

zzzzzzzzzzzzzzzzzzzzzzzzzzzzzzzzzzzzzzzzzzzzzzzzzzzzzzzzzzzzzzzzzzzz

Methods:

1. Skewer each banana slice into a toothpick.

2. Arrange bananas in a parchment lined baking pan. Put the pan into the freezer for an hour.

3. Place chopped dark chocolates and oil in a double boiler, stirring constantly until completely melted, about 4-5 minutes.

4. Dip each banana piece into warm chocolate mixture. Place the bananas back onto the pan, sprinkle with chopped almonds, and freeze for 1 hour before serving.

26) Tasty Sweet Corn and Herbs Bowl

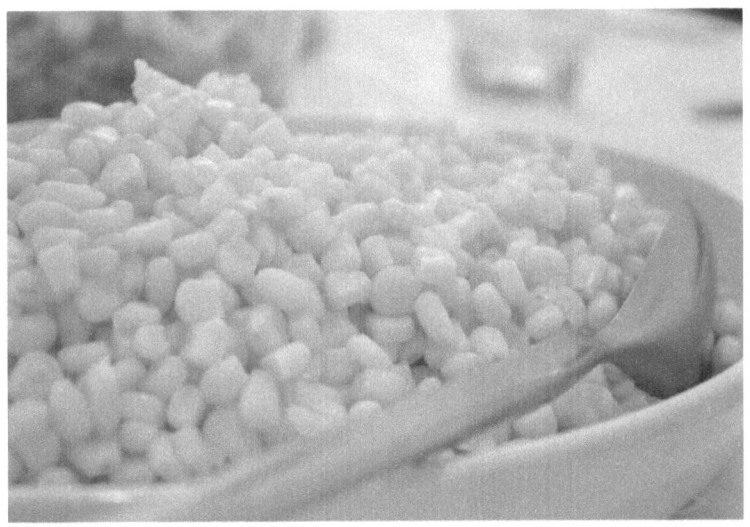

Sweet corn is not only tasty but also very healthy. It is loaded with vitamin C, manganese and dietary fiber, which are helpful as you prepare for giving birth. The crunchy, sweet summer veggie is also rich in B-vitamins and healthy carbohydrates. Mixing sweet corn with the finest herbs will make it even tastier and healthier. So, what are you waiting for? Try this recipe for a refreshing, easy-to-prepare meal.

Yield: 4

Preparation Time: 45 Minutes

Ingredient List:

- 4 corn on the cob, boiled and kernels sliced from the cob
- 3 ½ oz. red rice, cooked according to package directions
- 5 oz. quinoa, cooked according to package instructions
- 3 ½ oz. bulgur wheat, soaked in hot water for 20 minutes
- ½ cup mint leaves, coarsely chopped
- ½ cup flat leaf parsley, coarsely chopped
- ½ cup coriander leaves, coarsely chopped
- ½ cup basil leaves, coarsely chopped

For the dressing:

- 3 Tbsp. olive oil
- 2 cloves garlic, crushed
- 1 tsp. dried chili flakes
- Juice and zest of 2 limes

zzzzzzzzzzzzzzzzzzzzzzzzzzzzzzzzzzzzzzzzzzzzzzzzzzzzzzzzzzzzzzzzzzzz

Methods:

1. Combine cooked rice, quinoa, bulgar wheat, corn kernels and herbs in a large bowl. Set aside.

2. In a small bowl, combine the ingredients for the dressing. Pour over mixed grains and herbs.

3. Garnish with whole mint and coriander leaves. Serve.

27) Roast Turkey Breast with Herbs

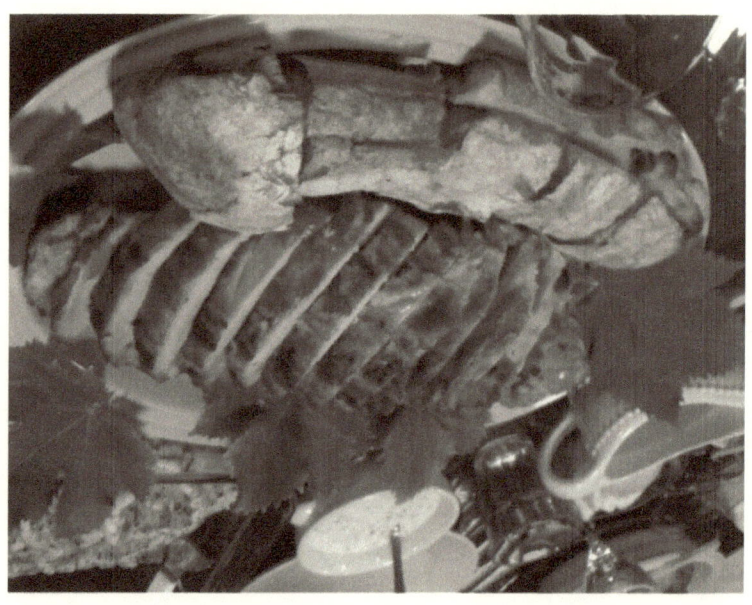

No fat protein is very helpful during pregnancy. That makes turkey an ideal meat choice when you need to beef up with protein to prepare for the upcoming baby delivery. Just make sure you stay away from deli turkey meats. Listeria, a bacteria that could cause harm to your yet-to-be-born child, may lurk in the shadows of deli counters. You must also heed the red-light warning about rotisserie turkey that is just being stocked in refrigerated cases. For this recipe, however, you are going to roast your turkey breast at about 325°F for almost 2 hours. That would erase all the potential risks of bacteria exposure and make you enjoy your meal worry-free.

Yield: 6

Preparation Time: 160 Minutes

Ingredient List:

- 1 whole turkey breast, bone in (about 7 lbs.)
- 3 cloves garlic, minced
- 1 Tbsp. of fresh rosemary leaves, chopped
- 1 Tbsp. fresh sage leaves, chopped
- 1 Tbsp. fresh thyme leaves, chopped
- 2 tsp. dry mustard
- 2 tsp. Kosher salt
- 2 Tbsp. extra virgin olive oil
- 2 Tbsp. lemon juice
- 1 cup dry white wine
- 1 tsp. freshly ground black pepper

ZZZZZZZZZZZZZZZZZZZZZZZZZZZZZZZZZZZZZZZZZZZZZZZZZZZZZZZZZZZZZZZZZ

Methods:

1. Preheat the oven to 325°F.

2. Place the turkey in a roasting rack, skin side up. Set aside.

3. In a bowl, mix garlic, mustard, herbs, olive oil and lemon juice. Season with salt and pepper, mixing until you make a paste.

4. Stuff half of the paste directly onto the loosen skin of the turkey breast. The remaining half should be spread evenly on the outer skin.

5. Pour wine into the bottom of the pan.

6. Roast until internal temperature reaches 165°F, about 105-120 minutes.

7. When done roasting, cover meat with aluminum foil and rest at room temperature for 15 minutes.

8. Slice and serve.

28) Honey-Glazed Brussel Sprouts

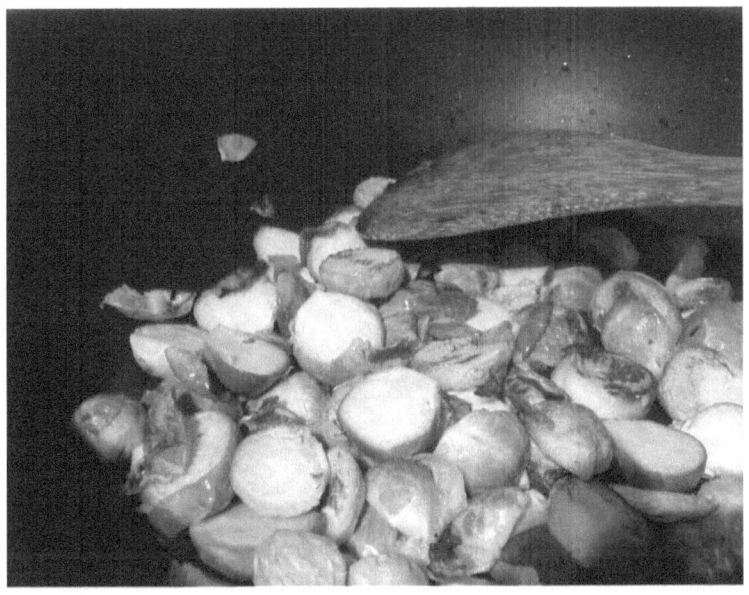

Brussel sprouts are a compact, flavorful veggie that pops into the mouth oozing with goodness and health benefits. They are nice to indulge in during pregnancy, especially while waiting for that big day when you are going to deliver a child. That's because they have B-vitamins, iron, vitamin C and fiber. Brussel sprouts are helpful in preventing birth defects, so you can deliver a normal and healthy baby. Just make sure you wash and cook the sprouts properly.

Yield: 4

Preparation Time: 25 minutes

Ingredient List:

- 1½ cup brussel sprouts, washed, trimmed, and halved
- 3 Tbsp. olive oil, divided
- 2 Tbsp. balsamic vinegar
- 2 tsp. honey
- ¾ cup kosher salt
- 1 tsp. ground black pepper

zzzzzzzzzzzzzzzzzzzzzzzzzzzzzzzzzzzzzzzzzzzzzzzzzzzzzzzzzzzzzzz

Methods:

1. Preheat oven to 425°F. Prepare a baking sheet lined with aluminum foil.

2. Mix brussel sprouts and 2 Tbsp. of olive oil in a bowl. Season with salt and pepper. Then, transfer onto prepared pan.

3. Roast until tender and caramelized, about 20 minutes.

4. Place roasted sprouts in a serving dish, toss with the remaining olive oil, honey, and balsamic vinegar. Coat evenly.

29) Lime and Mint Chicken BBQ

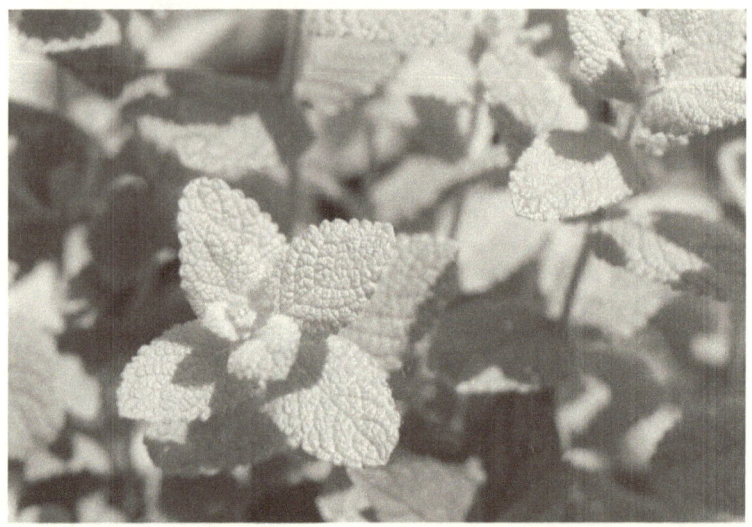

Skewers are a delight. When they are made of the good things, like chicken on this recipe, you will be able to guiltlessly indulge into them, even while you are pregnant. You will surely love the savory, garlicky, lemony, and minty flavors of these chicken thigh fillets on sticks.

Yield: 6

Preparation Time: 35 minutes

Ingredient List:

- 2½ lbs. chicken thigh fillets, cut into 2cm pieces
- Juice and rind of 2 limes
- ¼ cup fresh mint leaves
- ½ cup fresh coriander leaves
- 2 green chillies, halved, seeded, and chopped
- 2 cloves garlic, crushed
- ¼ cup light olive oil
- 2 Tbsp. water
- ½ cup Tzatziki

zzzzzzzzzzzzzzzzzzzzzzzzzzzzzzzzzzzzzzzzzzzzzzzzzzzzzzzzzzzzzz

Methods:

1. Mix lime rind, juice, chillies, garlic, coriander, mint, and oil in the food processor until smooth.

2. Coat chicken with processed marinade and place in the fridge for 20 minutes.

3. Place chicken into skewers, brush generously with marinade.

4. Cook chicken skewers in the grill over high fire, about 5 minutes or until cooked through.

5. Meanwhile, stir water onto Tzatziki.

6. Serve chicken skewers garnished with mint leaves and lime wedges along with the thickened sauce.

30) Salmon and Summer Veggies in Foil

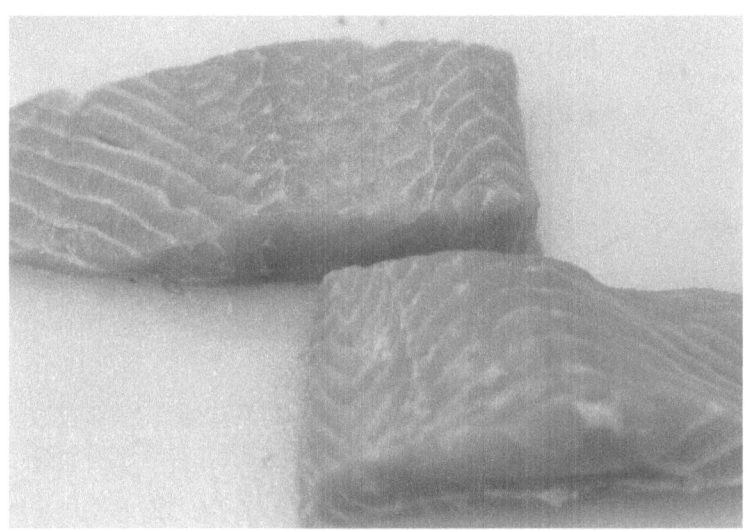

You can never have enough salmon at any stage of your pregnancy. During the trimester, when your energy requirements are unbelievably high, you need to nourish yourself with meals that are overflowing with vitamins and minerals. This salmon and veggie number is one great choice to include in your guidebook. It's a refreshing dish that you can prepare in a breeze.

Yield: 4

Preparation Time: 45 minutes

Ingredient List:

- 4 salmon fillets (5 oz.), skin on
- 2 yellow squash, sliced
- 2 zucchini, sliced
- 2 shallots, 1 sliced and 1 chopped
- 1 clove garlic, minced
- 2 tomatoes, diced
- 1 Tbsp. fresh thyme, chopped
- 3 tsp. dried oregano
- ½ tsp. dried marjoram
- 2½ Tbsp. olive oil
- 1½ Tbsp. lemon juice
- Salt and pepper to taste

ZZZZZZZZZZZZZZZZZZZZZZZZZZZZZZZZZZZZZZZZZZZZZZZZZZZZZZZZZZZZZZZ

Methods:

1. Preheat oven to 400°F.

2. Mix zucchini, yellow squash, sliced shallots, minced garlic and olive oil in a bowl. Season with salt and pepper.

3. Divide veggies into four. Place them in the center of a precut 17-inch length aluminum foil.

4. Season salmon fillets with salt and pepper before placing on top of veggies, drizzle with more olive oil and lemon juice.

5. Toss in tomatoes, diced shallots, thyme, oregano and marjoram with the remaining olive oil. Place on top of salmon.

6. Fold the ends of the foil to seal, arrange in a baking sheet, then cook in the oven for 25-30 minutes.

About the Author

A native of Albuquerque, New Mexico, Sophia Freeman found her calling in the culinary arts when she enrolled at the Sante Fe School of Cooking. Freeman decided to take a year after graduation and travel around Europe, sampling the cuisine from small bistros and family owned restaurants from Italy to Portugal. Her bubbly personality and inquisitive nature made her popular with the locals in the villages and when she finished her trip and came home, she had made friends for life in the places she had visited. She also came home with a deeper understanding of European cuisine.

Freeman went to work at one of Albuquerque's 5-star restaurants as a sous-chef and soon worked her way up to head chef. The restaurant began to feature Freeman's original dishes as specials on the menu and soon after, she began to write e-books with her recipes. Sophia's dishes mix local flavours with European inspiration making them irresistible to the diners in her restaurant and the online community.

Freeman's experience in Europe didn't just teach her new ways of cooking, but also unique methods of presentation. Using rich sauces, crisp vegetables and meat cooked to perfection, she creates a stunning display as well as a delectable dish. She has won many local awards for her cuisine and she continues to delight her diners with her culinary masterpieces.

Author's Afterthoughts

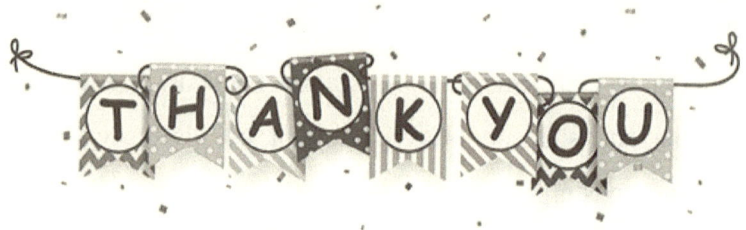

I want to convey my big thanks to all of my readers who have taken the time to read my book. Readers like you make my work so rewarding and I cherish each and every one of you.

Grateful cannot describe how I feel when I know that someone has chosen my work over all of the choices available online. I hope you enjoyed the book as much as I enjoyed writing it.

Feedback from my readers is how I grow and learn as a chef and an author. Please take the time to let me know your thoughts by leaving a review on Amazon so I and your fellow readers can learn from your experience.

My deepest thanks,

Sophia Freeman

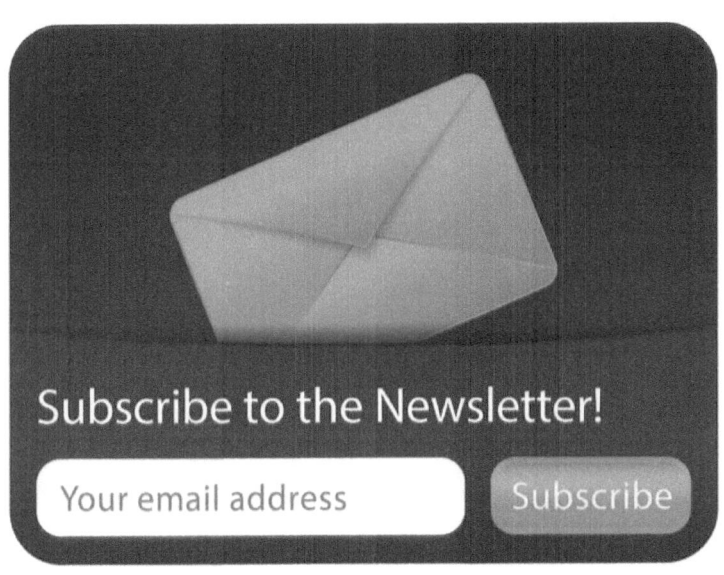

Subscribe to the Newsletter!

| Your email address | Subscribe |

https://sophia.subscribemenow.com/

✦ ✦ ✦ ★ ★ ★ ★ ★ ✦ ✦ ✦

www.ingramcontent.com/pod-product-compliance
Lightning Source LLC
Chambersburg PA
CBHW030403290526
45785CB00004B/1886